INTERMITTENT FASTING FOR MEN OVER 40:

Unlock the Power of Intermittent Fasting with These Tips for Men

JANET MARTINS

Contents

DISCLAIMER:

All content is provided as general information only, and should not be taken as medical advice or professional guidance. Please consult with a qualified healthcare provider if you have any questions or concerns about your individual situation.

INTRODUCTION

If you're a man over 40, you may be interested in intermittent fasting to improve your health. This type of fasting has been shown to have many benefits for men of this age, including weight loss, better blood sugar control, and improved heart health. In this blog post, we will discuss some tips for how to get started with intermittent fasting and make the most of its benefits.

If you're a man over 40 and looking to unlock the power of intermittent fasting, you're in luck. In this blog post, we will discuss some tips that will help you get started. Intermittent fasting can be a great way to improve your health and lose weight, but it can be challenging to get started if you need help knowing where to start. We will provide tips for getting started and advice on making intermittent fasting work for you.

PART 1

WHAT IS INTERMITTENT FASTING?

Intermittent fasting is an eating pattern that alternates between eating and fasting periods. It has been used to promote health, longevity, and weight loss for centuries. However, in recent years, intermittent fasting has become increasingly popular with men over 40 looking for an effective lifestyle change to improve their overall health and well-being.

Intermittent fasting is also known as time-restricted eating. It involves fasting for a set period each Day and consuming only calorie-free beverages during that window. Typically, this is done for 16 hours a day, leaving 8 hours to consume food. This approach helps promote fat loss, reduce inflammation, regulate blood sugar levels, and boost energy levels.

It is also important to note that intermittent fasting is not a diet. It is more of an eating pattern and lifestyle choice than a strict diet. That being said, it can still benefit those looking to lose weight or improve overall health.

Intermittent fasting means you don't eat for some time each day or week. Some popular approaches to intermittent fasting include:

- **Alternate-day fasting.** Eat a normal diet one Day and either completely fast or have one small meal (less than 500 calories) the next Day.
- **5:2 fasting.** Eat a normal diet five days a week and fast twice a week.
- **Daily time-restricted fasting.** Eat normally but only within an eight-hour

window each Day. For example, skip breakfast but eat lunch around noon and dinner by 8 pm.

According to a few studies, intermittent fasting may be just as efficient in promoting weight reduction as the traditional low-calorie diet. It makes sense, considering that cutting down on the calories you consume should assist you in achieving your weight loss goals.

Can intermittent fasting have any positive effects on your health? Obesity is linked to a higher risk of several disorders, including diabetes, sleep apnea, and even some forms of cancer. Reducing weight and increasing your physical activity may help reduce this risk. It seems that intermittent fasting is approximately as useful for treating these disorders as any other sort of diet that lowers the total number of calories consumed.

Some research suggests that intermittent fasting may be more beneficial than other diets for reducing inflammation and improving conditions associated with inflammation, such as:

- Alzheimer's disease
- Arthritis
- Asthma
- Multiple sclerosis
- Stroke

It's important to note that intermittent fasting can have unpleasant side effects, but they usually go away within a month. Side effects may include:

- Hunger
- Fatigue
- Insomnia
- Nausea
- Headaches

Intermittent fasting is safe for many people, but it's not for everyone. Skipping meals may not be the best way to manage your weight if you're pregnant or breastfeeding. If you have kidney stones, gastroesophageal reflux, diabetes, or other medical problems, talk with your doctor before starting intermittent fasting.

PATH TO IMPROVED HEALTH

A diet is not the same thing as intermittent fasting. It is more accurately described as an eating pattern, despite the fact that it may provide some of the same health advantages as a diet. It indicates that you abstain from eating within a certain window of time each Day (usually an extended period of time). After that, you consume food at a different time of Day each Day (usually a smaller period of time). You are allowed to consume drinks that do not contain calories while you are fasting. Some examples of these beverages include water, black coffee, and unsweetened tea.

An eating schedule refers to the way that each Day is split between periods of fasting and eating. The 16:8 schedule is one of the most often used and straightforward ones. This indicates that you will abstain from food for a period of 16 hours and consume all of your meals over a period of 8 hours. For instance, you may want to abstain from food and drink from 7 pm to 11 am the following Day. After that, between the hours of 11 am and 7 pm, you would have a nutritious lunch and supper. After 7 o'clock in the evening, you wouldn't be allowed to eat again until 11 o'clock the following morning. This is but one instance among many more. You have the flexibility to choose any 16-hour and 8-hour chunk of time that will fit with your schedule the best. Yet, it is essential to have a consistent time frame for eating every Day.

Other types of intermittent fasting include the 18:6 schedule (during which time you go without food for 18 hours and then eat normally for 6), as well as alternate days. On alternate days, you will abstain from food for twenty-four hours, then have a nutritious diet for twenty-four hours, and finally, you will fast for twenty-four hours. This timetable will continue to follow the pattern of having every other Day off. Another such timetable would be 5:2. This is the practice of abstaining from food on two days each week while maintaining a regular, nutritious diet for the other five days. On the days when you are supposed to be fasting, you are permitted to have a single meal consisting of between 500 and 600 calories. This is a little departure from the standard schedule.

HOW INTERMITTENT FASTING WORKS

Your metabolic rate will change after you have abstained from food for at least 12 hours. The process by which your body converts the fuel from the foods and beverages you consume into usable energy is called your metabolic system. The majority of the time, the sugar known as glucose is where your body gets its supply of energy from. Glucose can be found in the foods and beverages that you consume on a regular basis. Because you are consuming food and liquid on such a regular basis, your body is able to keep its glucose level stable when you eat three meals throughout the Day.

On the other hand, if you go without food for more than 12 hours, the glucose levels in your body will begin to drop since you won't be eating as regularly. When your body does not have access to the glucose that it needs for energy, it will draw energy from the fat that is stored in your body. When anything like this takes place, the fatty acids that are already present in your body are absorbed into your circulation. They result in the production of a chemical known as ketones. After then, your body makes use of the ketones as a source of energy. This phenomenon is referred to as a metabolic switch. Your body is transitioning away from using glucose and toward using ketones.

It's possible that you'll shed some pounds if your body starts running on ketones rather than fat. On the other hand, although you may not notice it, ketones may also be having a beneficial effect on the organs and cells of your body.

The advantages of intermittent fasting require that you abstain from food for a period of at least 12 hours. This is the amount of time it takes for your body to go from using glucose as a source of energy to utilizing fat instead. In addition, it will take some time for your body to adjust to the new eating plan that you will be following. So, you shouldn't anticipate instant results. It's possible that it will take anywhere from two to four weeks before you see or feel any results.

HEALTH BENEFITS OF INTERMITTENT FASTING

While researchers are still studying intermittent fasting, some research has shown it offers some health benefits. For starters, it's common to lose weight when following intermittent fasting. That's because your body is using fat, not glucose as its energy source. Additionally, if you make wise food choices when you do eat, you're likely eating fewer calories than before you started intermittent fasting. If you add exercise to the mix, it's a great combination for not only weight loss, but also improved health benefits. Intermittent fasting may help people who have cardiovascular disease, neurological disorders, and some cancers. Intermittent fasting may also help lower your bad cholesterol and improve symptoms of arthritis.

Be sure to talk with your doctor before you begin intermittent fasting. They will help you decide if it's a good fit for you. They will consider your current health, medicines, and health history when making their recommendation. If you have certain chronic health problems such as diabetes or heart disease, you may need to adjust or monitor your eating patterns.

PART 2:

BENEFITS OF INTERMITTENT FASTING FOR MEN OVER 40

- Weight loss
- Improvements in blood sugar
- Improvements in high blood pressure
- Lowered cholesterol
- Whole-body detoxification
- Reduction in oxidative stress and inflammation

That said, it's important to note that while there is recent research highlighting the short-term benefits of IF for weight loss and overall health, the long-term effects are unclear.

More evidence is needed on the long-term benefits before it can be prescribed for clinical use. Therefore, the best health strategy is to develop a healthy eating routine that works for your lifestyle while also incorporating regular exercise.

It's also important to note that you should always speak with a healthcare professional before engaging in a long-term diet change. And if you have a history of eating disorders or take certain medication, IF isn't recommended.

Lower risk of type 2 diabetes

IF can improve insulin sensitivity, reduce insulin resistance, lower blood sugar, and decrease fasting insulin levels, reducing your risk of developing type 2 diabetes.

Lower inflammation

Inflammation builds up in our bodies and can lead to many chronic health conditions, like high blood pressure or cardiovascular disease.

According to some studies, IF can reduce inflammation.

A healthier heart

By lowering things like LDL cholesterol, triglycerides, inflammation, blood sugar, and insulin resistance, intermittent fasting supports our heart health.

A smarter, stronger brain

Even your brain benefits—some studies show that IF helps promote neuroplasticity and makes the brain hardier to injury and disease.

MAKE IF WORK FOR YOU

1. Plan your grocery shop for the entire week.
2. Optimise food quality by fueling with predominantly whole foods (fruits, vegetables, beans, lean proteins, and healthy fats) while avoiding sugars and refined grains.

3. Prepare your own comfort food. Having healthy snacks or sweets will minimize cravings for sugar and processed foods.

4. Avoid snacking late at night, while incorporating snacks rich in quality protein and dietary fiber between meals to help manage appetite.

5. Avoid sugary drinks and diet sodas.

6. Stick to lots of water, black coffee, or an americano within the fasting window.

7. Hydration is key during the fasting window to maximize whole-body detoxification.

Example 14:10 IF Day

10:00 am Fast Breaker: Banana Protein Smoothie

12:00 pm Meal 1: Breakfast Burrito

1:30 pm Snack: Chocolate Date Protein Balls

3:30 pm Meal 2: Pesto Chicken and Salad Wrap

6:30 pm Meal 3: Avocado and Sweet Potato Salmon

PART 3

GUIDELINES FOR STARTING AN INTERMITTENT FASTING PLAN

Find your deeper motivation

Say you start IF today. Imagine yourself a few months down the line.

What has improved in your life?

- Are you more comfortable in your body?
- Are you rocking that outfit you've always felt too self-conscious to wear?
- Are you standing taller, with a sense of confidence and pride?

- Are you moving better, your joints feeling less clunky?
- Do you have energy for days?
- Do you feel settled and easy in how you're eating?

Tap into that vision. Add color and clarity to it. Write it out, draw a picture, make a collage—do it anyhow you like.

A strong, vivid goal is a real ally, especially on tougher days.

Build your IF team

Speaking of allies, at SIMPLE we're always in your corner.

We're super experienced at intermittent fasting (and have a real soft spot for beginners).

Get started with our quiz and we'll walk the IF path with you, bringing ideas to inspire you, encouragement for the rough days, and support when you get stuck.

Be prepared

The early intermittent fasting phase can be a little rocky. Being prepared makes *so* much difference to whether you calmly ride out that stage with composure, or whether it reduces you to a flailing mess.

Here are the things to be ready for. In the first two weeks of your intermittent fasting plan, you will most likely feel:

- hungry
- irritable
- tired
- cold
- headachy
- a grumpy belly

At times you may even feel like this IF thing is too hard but hang in there. These feelings will pass, and there are things you can do to help yourself through them.

Choose your intermittent fasting plan

As a beginner, you're free to play around with various intermittent fasting schedules to find the one you like best.

Let's look at how each one works.

Intermittent fasting 16/8

On a 16/8 fasting schedule, you alternate between 16 hours of fasting and an 8-hour eating window.

This method simply extends the timeframe of the natural daily fast that happens when you're sleeping. You don't need to count calories, and you can set up the 8-hour eating window any way you want (yes, you *can* eat breakfast, and let nobody tell you otherwise!).

The warrior diet

The warrior diet is a 20-hour fast, followed by a 4-hour eating window.

You've probably done it once or twice by accident in your life, like that time you went to your friend's wedding and the food didn't show up for hours (even the balloons were looking delicious at that point).

But as a daily approach? Whether you could eat enough in that 4-hour window to satisfy all your nutritional needs is questionable. We're not gonna lie; it's a tough intermittent fasting schedule to start with for beginners.

The 5:2 diet

The 5:2 diet is a fasting plan where you eat as you usually would 5 days per week and eat just 500/600 calories on the other 2.

For some people, it's easier to restrict calories on just two days per week, compared to a daily fasting schedule like 16/8. But for others, a whole day with only 500/600 calories to bolster them causes too much hunger, fatigue, and stress.

Eat Stop Eat

Eat Stop Eat means eating as you normally would on day 1, then fasting until dinner on day 2. You'd eat at least one full meal every Day (and that meal is your choice).

A 24-hour fast is a hefty undertaking, and at SIMPLE, we tend not to recommend it. It can make it pretty challenging to meet all your nutritional needs which, over time, could add up to some serious nutrient deficiencies.

Alternate day fasting

Alternate-day fasting is similar to 5:2 but somewhat more intense: You fast every other Day, and, on those fasting days, you eat 500/600 calories. This alternating pattern makes for three or four fasting days each week.

That's a lot of fasting, huh? Because of that, this might not be the ideal fasting approach for beginners. If this weekly on/off style appeals to you, 5:2 would be a good starting place.

Water fasting

Water fasting entails going 24-72 hours drinking only water and going completely without food.

It's an approach we don't recommend here at SIMPLE unless you're going to do it with medical supervision.

PART 4:

COMMON INTERMITTENT FASTING MISTAKES TO AVOID

Mistake 1: Not Choosing The Right Intermittent Fasting Plan

Taking a one-size-fits-all approach to intermittent fasting is one of the biggest mistakes people make. Not everyone's body responds the same way to fasting. What works for some may not work for you.

That's why it's important to find a plan that fits your lifestyle, schedule, and goals. It's important to note that there are many different types of intermittent fasting plans to choose from.

- **16/8** – This is the most common type of IF. You fast for 16 hours, usually overnight, and eat within an 8-hour window.

- **24-Hour Fast** – This is exactly what it sounds like. You fast for 24 hours, usually once or twice a week.

- **5:2 Diet** – On 2 non-consecutive days of the week, you eat 500-600 calories. The other 5 days you eat normally.

- **Alternate Day Fasting** – On fasting days, you eat 25% of your normal caloric intake. On non-fasting days, you eat normally.

- **The Warrior Diet** – This is a 20-hour fast with a 4-hour eating window.

- **The Eat-Stop-Eat Method** – This is a 24-hour fast once or twice a week.

Why It's A Problem

Choosing a plan that's too strict or not well suited for your lifestyle is a recipe for disaster. You're more likely to cheat or give up altogether if you're constantly hungry or feeling deprived.

On the flip side, if you choose a plan that's too lax, you won't see the results you're looking for. In addition, you won't be pushing your body to its full potential.

How To Fix It

The best way to find the right intermittent fasting plan is to experiment with different methods until you find one that works for you. Start with a 16/8 split and see how you feel. You can also work in different length fasting windows on different days of the week according to your schedule – like 12/12 or 14/10 on days when 16/8 just doesn't fit or you don't feel up to it. If you're struggling with doing some type of fasting every Day, try a 24-hour fast or the 5:2 diet.

Remember, there is no one perfect plan. The key is finding one that you can stick to long-term without feeling deprived or restricted.

Mistake 2: Not Considering Your Lifestyle

The most successful lifestyle changes are the ones that are easiest to stick to. That's why it's important to consider your lifestyle when choosing an intermittent fasting plan.

There are several aspects of your lifestyle that determine whether a particular fasting plan will work for you:

- **Your schedule** – If you have a busy lifestyle with little time for meals, an 8-hour eating window every Day may not be feasible.
- **Your dietary restrictions and preferences** – Some fasting plans allow for more flexibility than others.
- **The number of meals you eat per Day** – If you're used to eating 3 meals a

day, going to an all-day fast may be too difficult.

- **How active you are** – active people require more energy and need to eat more often than sedentary people.

- **Your social life** – If you have a busy social life, avoiding restaurants and social gatherings may be difficult.

Why It's A Problem

Not considering your lifestyle when choosing an intermittent fasting plan can make it very difficult to stick to. You're more likely to cheat or give up if you're constantly struggling to fit fasting into your already busy schedule.

How To Fix It

The best way to fix this mistake is to choose an intermittent fasting plan that fits your lifestyle. Bear in mind that IF is all about time-restricted eating, so any plan that allows you to eat within a set timeframe will work.

If you have a busy lifestyle, try the 16/8 method or the warrior diet. If you have an active social life, you may find it easier to do a longer fast once or twice a week on days when you don't have social engagements, like the 24-hour fast or the alternate-day fasting method.

Mistake 3: Not Eating Enough When You Break Your Fast

People often confuse IF with dieting. This leads to the common misconception that you should eat very little during your eating window. This is not only ineffective, but it can also be dangerous.

In reality, there's a huge difference between the two. IF restricts the time you eat, while dieting restricts the type and amount of food you eat. The whole point of IF is to give your body a break from digesting food.

Why It's A Problem

Underneath all the fat you're trying to lose, your body has lean muscle. This muscle is important because it helps you burn calories, even when you're resting, plus you need it to do all the daily activities of life. When you don't eat enough on fasting days, your body starts to break down this muscle for energy.

This not only slows down your metabolism, but it can also cause muscle wasting and fatigue.

Undereating also makes you more likely to binge eat later. This can offset any weight loss you've achieved and make it harder to stick to your plan in the long run.

How To Fix It

The most effective solution for correcting this error is to ensure that you consume a sufficient amount of food within the time allotted to eating. How can you determine how much is sufficient?

Calculating the amount of energy and protein that your body requires based on individual circumstances, activity levels, and objectives is a reasonable rule of thumb to follow. This will assist in preventing the loss of muscle and will keep your metabolism going strong.

Spread the caloric intake out throughout the period of your eating window, which should consist of anywhere from two to four meals depending on the sort of fasting you are undergoing.

There are a lot of calorie calculators available online, and you may use one of them to figure out how many calories you need to consume each Day.

Using the hand-size approach is still another alternative. Consuming a portion of protein equal to the size of your palm, a portion of vegetables equal to the size of your fist, and a quantity of carbs equal to the size of your cupped hand at each meal is required.

Mistake 4: Eating Too Much When You Break Your Fast

Hunger after a fast is completely normal, but eating too much can quickly offset any weight loss you've achieved. This is another common mistake that people make when they start intermittent fasting.

The hormone ghrelin is responsible for making you feel hungry, and it's also responsible for increasing your appetite after a fast. When you overeat, ghrelin spikes and makes you even hungrier than you were before. This can quickly lead to weight gain and stalled progress.

Why It's A Problem

Overeating negates the benefits of IF and can lead to weight gain. It also makes it harder to stick to your fasting plan in the long run.

How To Fix It

Start by eating a small, nutritious meal when you break your fast. This will help stave off hunger without overeating. Here are some nutritious, filling meals you can use to break your fast:

- Yogurt with chia seeds
- Bone or vegetable broth
- A small salad with grilled chicken
- A veggie omelet
- A green smoothie
- A bowl of fruit

You can also try drinking a glass of water or herbal tea before meals to help you feel more full.

And if you're still struggling, try eating more protein- and fiber-rich foods. These nutrients are known for their ability to help control hunger and promote satiety.

If you're still feeling hungry after your first meal, wait 20-30 minutes before having a second. This will give your body time to register that it's full.

Mistake 5: Choosing The Wrong Foods During Your Eating Window

The eating window is a period of time during which you are free to consume any foods you want. And even while there are no restrictions on what you may or cannot eat, there are certainly meals that are superior to others.

Your insulin levels will surge and you will contribute to weight gain if you consume ultra-processed junk food, sugary beverages, and refined carbohydrates. On the other hand, eating entire foods such as veggies, whole grains, lean protein, and healthy fats will help you enhance your health while also assisting you in shedding excess pounds.

Why It's A Problem

Consuming junk food that has been processed nullifies the positive effects of intermittent fasting and may lead to weight gain. Also, it may have a role in the development of other health issues, such as diabetes, cardiovascular disease, and high blood pressure.

Additionally, your body reacts differently to meals that have been excessively processed as opposed to those that are in their natural state. Since they are digested more slowly, whole foods do not induce the same jump in insulin levels that highly processed meals do because they do not include any added sugars. Consuming foods in their natural, unprocessed state may assist in weight loss and enhance overall health.

How To Fix It

Eliminate ultra-processed junk food from your diet and replace it with whole foods. Here are some healthy, whole foods you can include during your eating window:

- Vegetables
- Fruit
- Lean protein
- Nuts and seeds
- Whole grains
- Healthy fats

Here are some foods that you should avoid:

- Sugary drinks
- Refined carbs e.g. white bread, pastries
- Processed meats e.g. bacon, sausage
- Junk food e.g. candy, cake, cookies

Mistake 6: Not Staying Hydrated

Water is essential for weight loss, regardless of whether you're fasting or not. Drinking plenty of water while fasting helps you feel fuller and less prone to cravings. Furthermore, your body functions better when it's well-hydrated.

Why It's A Problem

Not staying hydrated can lead to dehydration, which can cause a slew of health problems. These include:

- Headache
- Dizziness
- Fatigue
- Nausea
- Constipation

Furthermore, dehydration can make it harder to lose weight. This is because water helps to flush out toxins and keep your metabolism working properly.

How To Fix It

Drink at least 8 glasses of water a day, especially during your fasting periods. You can also drink other beverages like unsweetened green tea or herbal teas.

While unsweetened black coffee is okay in moderation, caffeine can dehydrate you. So make sure to drink an extra glass of water for every cup of coffee you have.

Mistake 7: You're Unknowingly Breaking Your Fast

Many people don't understand what a clean fast means. A clean fast, which is what you're expected to do during your fasting window, means not consuming anything but water, black coffee, and unsweetened tea.

It's important to be aware of what you're drinking during your fast because many common drinks contain hidden calories and carbs.

Foods that are close to zero calories or labeled "diet" or "zero-calorie" are often full of artificial sweeteners, some of which can break your fast.

Why It's A Problem

Your fast will be considered broken, and the advantages of intermittent fasting will be nullified if you consume anything other than water, black coffee, and unsweetened tea while you are in your fasting window. This may cause you to feel frustrated and disheartened, and it may even drive you to give up on the intermittent fasting strategy completely.

In addition, in order to get the full advantages of fasting, one must go without eating for a lengthy period of time. Ketosis and autophagy are two examples of these benefits. Thus, if you often break your fast, you may never have the chance to experience these advantages.

How To Fix It

If you're not sure whether a drink is allowed during your fast, check the ingredients list. If it contains any sugar or artificial sweeteners, it's best to avoid it.

Look out for products containing:

- **Sugar or sugar alcohols** – common names include sucrose, fructose, maltose, lactose, xylitol, and erythritol
- **Artificial sweeteners** – common names include aspartame, saccharin, and sucralose
- **Natural sweeteners** – common names include honey, agave nectar, and maple syrup

Mistake 8: You're Not Exercising

Whether you're trying to lose weight or improve your health, exercise is important. Exercise helps to increase your metabolism, burn calories, and improve insulin sensitivity. All of these things are beneficial for weight loss and improved health.

Why It's A Problem

Some of the advantages of fasting will be lost if you don't take advantage of them by engaging in physical activity while you're doing it. Both elevating your metabolism and increasing the number of calories you burn via activity are essential components of successful weight reduction.

Those who fast often also experience a reduction in their muscle mass. Because of this, when you go without food for an extended period of time, your body will start to break down muscle tissue for energy. This may cause a reduction in muscle mass as well as a slowdown in the pace at which your body burns calories.

You can assist avoid this by engaging in regular strength training, which can also help you grow muscle, which, in the long run, may make it easier for you to maintain a healthy weight.

How To Fix It

Intermittent fasting is not an excuse to avoid exercise. In fact, exercising while fasting can help you burn more fat and improve your health.

Aim for at least 30 minutes of moderate-intensity exercise most days of the week. This could include walking, biking, swimming, or lightweight training.

If you're new to exercise:

- Start slow and gradually increase your intensity and duration over time.
- Time your workouts around your eating windows. This will help make sure you have the energy to fuel your workouts.
- Don't overdo it. Overtraining can counteract the benefits of fasting and actually make you gain weight.
- Stay hydrated before, during, and after your workouts. Drink plenty of water and avoid sugary sports drinks.

Mistake 9: You're Not Sleeping Enough

Getting enough sleep is important for both your physical and mental health. Not only does it help you recover from exercise, but it also helps to regulate your appetite.

Why It's A Problem

The hormone ghrelin is produced in greater quantities by the body of a person who does not get enough sleep. This hormone causes a rise in hunger as well as a desire for meals that are rich in calories.

Another factor that might contribute to weight gain is insufficient sleep. This is at least partially due to the fact that it may interfere with your body's capacity to manage the levels of insulin and blood sugar.

How To Fix It

Aim for 7-9 hours of quality sleep per night. If you have trouble sleeping, try some of these tips:

- Create a bedtime routine and stick to it

- Avoid caffeine and alcohol before bed

- Exercise regularly

- Keep your bedroom cool, dark, and quiet

Mistake 10: You're Not Being Patient

Weight loss is a slow process. It can take weeks or even months to see results. This can be frustrating, especially if you're used to seeing results quickly.

Even if you're not getting into IF for weight loss, most of its benefits come with time.

Why It's A Problem

It's easy to feel like giving up when you're not seeing the outcomes you were hoping for from your efforts. This may cause yo-yo dieting, which in turn can lead to weight gain.

A cycle of losing and gaining weight, sometimes known as "yo-yo dieting." It is hazardous to your health and may make it more difficult for you to shed weight in the years to come.

The irritation that you feel when you are not seeing results quickly enough might cause you to make additional errors, such as not eating enough or exercising too much.

How To Fix It

Be patient and give your body time to adjust. Remember that weight loss is a slow process and can take weeks or even months to see results.

Focus on other potential benefits of intermittent fasting, such as improved mental health, energy levels, and digestion.

If you're struggling with your weight, seek professional help. A dietitian or nutritionist can help create a plan that's right for you and help you stay on track.

PART 5:

TIPS FOR STICKING WITH INTERMITTENT FASTING

Intermittent fasting has lately gained a lot of popularity among fitness enthusiasts and dieters. It is an effective way to lose weight and stay healthy and fit. Intermittent fasting is all about timed eating, where you have to eat in a fixed time interval and abstain from having anything in the remaining hours. It is quite a simple diet trend, but embarking on any new journey can be intimidating. So, here are four tricks that can make Intermittent fasting easier for you.

Take it as a new habit

While the majority of us are used to eating three times each Day, changing the times at which we eat might make us feel uncomfortable. Even if you are not hungry, you will inexplicably have the want to eat something at lunch or breakfast even if you won't really be hungry at those times. While this may be difficult at first, consider it the beginning of a new routine. Any new routine requires a period of time for our body to adjust and get acclimated to it. You have to get yourself psychologically ready for the kind of change that is coming. It is going to be challenging at first, therefore it is important that you continually remind yourself why you have decided to follow this diet and that you remain steadfast in your choice. Adjusting to any new trend in nutrition is more of a mental challenge than a physical one.

Be strategic

During the first few days of your fast, you may find that you wake up in the morning feeling very hungry. This is quite normal. It's possible that you'll have an overwhelming want to chew on anything at all. Be aware of what you consume in the hours leading up to the beginning of your fast in order to avoid putting yourself in a precarious position. Consume an adequate amount of fiber, protein, and whole grains, and above all else, ensure that you drink lots of water. Consuming nutritious and filling meals prior to beginning your fast can help you feel fuller for a greater portion of the time that you will be fasting.

Motivate yourself

Take it as a challenge and you will be easily able to sail through it. If you feel sluggish in the beginning, of course, you will find it difficult. If you are excited about the idea of fasting, it will be a little easier. Convince yourself that you will feel better after doing it.

Keep experimenting

When it comes to intermittent fasting, there is no hard and fast rule; thus, you should make little adjustments to see what works best for you. It is not a given that what is successful for other people will also be successful for you. While abstaining from food for 18 hours might be beneficial for some individuals, you should not do this if you are unable to do so successfully. If you feel that 12 hours is the right amount for you, then stay with it.

TAKING CONTROL OF YOUR HEALTH WITH INTERMITTENT FASTING

If you're a man over 40, intermittent fasting can be a great way to improve your health and wellness. It's an effective lifestyle choice that can help you boost energy levels, maintain a healthy weight, and even lower your risk of chronic diseases like heart disease and diabetes.

With intermittent fasting, you cycle between periods of eating and not eating. This has many positive effects on your body, including improved metabolism, increased energy levels, and better concentration. In addition to these benefits, research shows that men may also see improvements in their cholesterol levels and blood pressure when following an intermittent fasting regimen.

While there are several different types of intermittent fasting methods such as time-restricted feeding or the 5:2 diet, the 16:8 method is typically recommended for men over 40. This involves fasting for up to 16 hours and only eating during an 8-hour window. During this time you can still eat a balanced diet of nutritious foods like lean proteins, healthy fats, and plenty of fruits and vegetables.

Intermittent fasting may require some adjustments to your daily routine, but once you get used to it, you'll likely find that it's easy to stick with. Plus, the long-term health benefits make intermittent fasting an effective and sensible choice for many men over 40. So why not give it a try? You just might be surprised at how much better you feel!

Fasting has been around for centuries and with the help of modern science, we now know that it's a great way to take control of your health. So if you're a man over 40 looking for an effective lifestyle choice to improve your well-being and help protect against chronic diseases, intermittent fasting may just be the perfect solution.

CONCLUSION

Intermittent fasting is an effective lifestyle choice for men over 40, offering tremendous health benefits. Studies have been conducted that show intermittent fasting can lead to improved overall health, increased energy levels, and a healthier weight. This type of fasting also helps to reduce the risk of chronic illnesses such as diabetes, cardiovascular disease, and stroke. It can even help improve mental clarity and focus. Intermittent fasting may take some getting used to, but with proper planning and dedication, it is definitely a practice worth exploring!

www.ingramcontent.com/pod-product-compliance
Lightning Source LLC
Chambersburg PA
CBHW071025260726
48662CB00024B/2010

Jane began to unravel the layers of trauma and negative self-talk that had been holding her back for so long while working with a therapist. Deep breathing and cognitive-behavioral therapy were among the methods she acquired for managing her depression and anxiety. She also joined a support group, where she got to know other people who were going through the same struggles.

Jane wanted to give up at times because it wasn't easy. Be that as it may, she continued to, not set in stone to defeat the devils inside herself. She began to notice small changes in her mood and behavior over time. She stopped relying on alcohol and drugs as a means of coping and began to feel more confident in social settings.

Jane is significantly better off than she was previously. She is proud of the person she has become because she has rebuilt her life. She is aware that the demons within her will always be present, but she has learned to control them and lead a happy life. She trusts that by sharing her story, she can motivate other people who are battling with comparable issues to realize that they are in good company and that there is consistent trust for recuperation.

Mark's Story: Fighting for Life Against the Darkness

The story of Mark is one of perseverance and resolve in the face of overwhelming darkness. He attempted suicide after struggling with depression and anxiety as a teenager. He was treated and put in the hospital, but he still felt like he was losing the fight against the darkness inside of him.

Mark tried to manage his depression and anxiety on his own for years, but he had trouble finding his life's purpose or meaning. He went to liquor and medications as a method for adapting, which just compounded the situation. When he lost his job, his home, and his sense of self-worth, he hit rock bottom.

Mark realized at this point that he required assistance. He talked to a therapist and started working on his problems with his mental health. He also started making positive changes in his life, like getting sober, exercising regularly, and getting back in touch with people he cared about.

Mark continued to struggle with depression and anxiety despite these efforts. He was once more in a pit of despair, but this time he refused to give up. He kept on looking for help and backing, in any event, when it seemed like there was no reason to have some hope.

Mark began to notice incremental changes in his mood and behavior over time. He found joy in simple things like spending time with loved ones or going for a walk in the woods, and he started to feel like his life had a purpose.

Mark is a shining example of what it means to fight against the darkness for life today. He has rebuilt his life from the ground up and is now a mental health advocate who promotes the importance of seeking mental health care. He trusts that by sharing his story, he can motivate other people who are battling with comparative issues to realize that they are in good company and that there is general trust for recuperation.

Sarah's Story: Surviving the Storm

The story of Sarah is one of perseverance in the face of overwhelming hardship. She was abused and neglected as a child, resulting in feelings of isolation, anxiety, and depression. She frequently had the impression that she was constantly caught in a storm of emotions and struggled to find a sense of safety or security in her life.

Sarah used alcohol and drugs to deal with her pain as she got older. She fell into a downward spiral after developing an addiction and was unable to break free from the cycle of self-destructive behavior and addiction.

Sarah didn't realize that she needed assistance until she reached rock bottom. She contacted a rehab facility and began working on her recovery. Meditation, therapy, and exercise were among the healthy coping strategies she picked up to deal with her emotions and trauma. She also joined a support group, where she connected with people who were going through the same problems as her.

Sarah persevered despite the difficulties. She began slowly, one day at a time, to rebuild her life. She got a new line of work, made new companions, and, surprisingly, began to seek after her interests and interests. She realized that she was capable of overcoming the storm within herself and that she was more powerful than she had ever imagined.

Today, Sarah is a survivor whose story of courage and tenacity serves as an inspiration to others. She works to spread the word about how important it is for people who are dealing with trauma or addiction to get help and is an advocate for mental health and addiction recovery. She is aware that the internal storm may never completely pass, but she has learned how to weather it and come out the other side stronger.

Chapter 2: Conquering Anxiety

Regardless of age, gender, or background, anxiety is a common emotion that can affect anyone. Anxiety can be helpful in some situations, like getting ready for a job interview or a big presentation, but excessive and persistent anxiety can make a person's life miserable. It can affect their relationships, their ability to function normally, and even their physical health.

Fortunately, there are numerous approaches to anxiety management. CBT, mindfulness meditation, exercise, and medication are all examples of these. We'll look at some of the best ways to get over anxiety in this chapter.

Cognitive-Behavioral Therapy (CBT)
CBT is a form of treatment that focuses on altering unfavorable thought patterns and behaviors that cause worry. Working with a clinician to recognize these habits and learn how

to substitute them with more positive and productive methods of thinking is part of the process. CBT is often used as a first-line therapy for anxiety conditions because it is extremely successful.

Mindfulness Meditation

Focusing your concentration on the current instant and becoming more conscious of your thoughts and emotions without judgment is what mindfulness meditation entails. It helps decrease anxious symptoms and increase general well-being. Mindfulness meditation comes in many varieties, including guided meditation, body scan meditation, and breathing meditation.

Exercise

Regular exercise can be a very effective strategy for lowering worry. Endorphins, which are natural chemicals that foster emotions of pleasure and well-being, are released as a result. Exercise can also aid in the reduction of muscular tension and the improvement of slumber, both of which can add to anxiety. It doesn't have to be anything strenuous; simply going for a stroll or practicing gentle yoga can be helpful.

Medication

Medication can be an effective aid in the treatment of anxiety, especially in those with significant symptoms. Anxiety medicine can be given in a variety of forms, including selective serotonin reuptake inhibitors (SSRIs), benzodiazepines, and beta-blockers. Working carefully with a healthcare practitioner to identify the best medicine and dose for your specific requirements is critical.

Self-Care

Self-care is an essential part of worry management. It entails attending to your bodily and mental requirements, such as getting enough sleep, consuming a wholesome diet, participating in enjoyable activities, and spending time with loved ones. Setting limits, saying no to things that cause excessive tension, and addressing your requirements are all examples of self-care.

To summarize, anxiety can be a difficult feeling to beat, but with the proper tactics and support, it is possible to overcome it. Remember that there is no one-size-fits-all strategy to cognitive-behavioral treatment, awareness meditation, exercise, medicine, or self-care. The important thing is to figure out what works best for you.

David's Story: Finding Freedom from Fear

David's is a tale of bravery and resilience in the face of adversity. David had always been a timid and reticent person, and his dread of public speaking and social encounters only developed as he got older. He struggled to make acquaintances, attend social events, and even speak up in class. This dread had a significant effect on both his personal and professional life, preventing him from achieving his ambitions and objectives.

David recognized the importance of breaking free from the grasp of dread that was preventing him from living his best life. He resolved to seek assistance and started working with an anxiety condition specialist psychiatrist. David learned to recognize the underlying reasons for his dread and to create coping techniques to control his worry through counseling.

One of David's most important turning moments was when he resolved to confront his dread of public speaking. He had always avoided situations in which he had to talk in front of others, but he realized that if he wanted to advance in his job, he needed to conquer this anxiety.

He joined a public speaking organization and started rehearsing talks in front of a tiny audience. Although he was initially apprehensive, he eventually gained confidence in speaking in public.

David's increased confidence permeated other aspects of his existence. He started taking more chances and pursuing his interests without dread of failure or disapproval. He met new people and started to appreciate social gatherings. As he became more open and talkative, his interactions with his family and colleagues improved.

David's path to overcoming anxiety was not simple, but it was worthwhile. He found that by confronting his anxieties and stepping outside of his comfort zone, he could accomplish his objectives and live a better, more satisfying existence. His tale can serve as an encouragement to others who are dealing with worry and dread, demonstrating that it is possible to surmount these obstacles and achieve personal development and achievement.

Samantha's Story: Learning to Live with the Unthinkable

Samantha's tale is a potent testimony to the human spirit's resilience in the face of unfathomable disaster. Samantha was identified with a severe type of brain cancer at the age of 28 that required urgent and extensive therapy. Samantha stayed optimistic and resolved to battle for her life despite the chances stacked against her.

Samantha endured numerous operations, bouts of chemotherapy, and radiation treatment over the next few months. She felt the bodily and mental toll these therapies had on her body, but she refused to give up. Samantha took courage from her religion, her family, and her resolve throughout it all.

Samantha learned to negotiate a new world as she battled for her life, one in which she would have to live with the unpredictability of her future and the possibility of recurrence. She battled with the dread and anxiousness that this new reality brought, but she refused to let it define her.

Instead, Samantha channeled her energy into assisting others who were going through similar difficulties. She became a cancer researcher and champion, telling her experience and giving hope to others battling for their lives. Samantha discovered a new mission in life through her activism work, one that gave her courage and optimism even in the darkest of times.

Samantha's path was not without ups and downs, but she never wavered in her resolve to live a complete and fulfilling life. She learned to accept the difficulties and doubts that life threw at her, viewing them as chances for personal growth and development.

Samantha is now a source of optimism for others who are experiencing similar difficulties. Her tale is a potent lesson that no matter what life tosses at us, we can conquer even the most insurmountable hurdles.

Michael's Story: Overcoming Panic and Paralysis

Michael's tale is one of perseverance and courage in the face of hardship. He suffered from panic episodes and immobility, which left him feeling exhausted and unable to progress forward in his life.

Michael had suffered from worry and melancholy for many years. He had always been a delicate and thoughtful person, but his worry started to take over his life as he got older. He'd frequently wake up in the middle of the night, unable to collect his breath or quiet his rushing thoughts.

Michael attempted everything to alleviate his worry, from meditation and awareness to medicine and counseling. But no matter what he did, he couldn't get rid of the dread and terror that seemed to be hovering just beneath the surface.

Michael determined enough was enough one day. He was sick of feeling imprisoned and helpless, and he was resolved to reclaim his life. He began by establishing modest objectives for himself, such as going for a stroll or contacting a buddy. Every time he achieved one of these objectives, he felt a feeling of satisfaction and achievement, which served to boost his confidence.

Michael started to gain a better grasp of his nervousness as he continued to work on himself. He learned to identify the factors that set off his panic episodes and created coping techniques for when they happened. He also learned to be gentler and more patient with himself, recognizing that conquering his worry would take time and work.

Michael's perseverance paid off over time. He was able to conquer his panic episodes and the immobility that had previously held him back. He began to feel more secure and in charge of his life, and he resumed the pursuit of his interests and goals.

Michael is now a bright model of what persistence and resolve can achieve. He has surmounted seemingly overwhelming hurdles and is now leading a complete and happy existence. His tale serves as a lesson that no matter how difficult the obstacles we confront appear to be, we can conquer them and accomplish our objectives with hard work and perseverance.

Chapter 3: Wrestling with Bipolar Disorder

Bipolar disorder, also known as manic-depressive disease, is a mental illness characterized by severe mood fluctuations, including periods of euphoria and sadness. These emotional changes can be strong and unexpected, making everyday life challenging for people with bipolar illness.

In this chapter, we will look at what bipolar disorder is, what its signs are, and how it impacts people who have it. We will also go over some of the therapies and coping techniques that can help people with bipolar disorder control their symptoms and live a better life.

What exactly is Bipolar Disorder?

Bipolar disease is a psychiatric illness that impacts about 2.8% of people in the United

States. It is marked by manic and melancholy bouts that differ in duration and severity.

Mania is characterized by excessive energy, exhilaration, and, frequently, recklessness. Individuals may experience increased activity, reduced need for sleep, rushing ideas, and heightened self-esteem during a euphoric phase. They may participate in hazardous behaviors such as excessive expenditures, drug misuse, and traveling recklessly.

Depression, on the other hand, is characterized by fatigue, sorrow, and despair. Individuals suffering from depression may experience emotions of worthlessness, trouble focusing, and changes in eating and sleep habits. They may also have suicidal ideas.

Bipolar disease is divided into three types: bipolar I, bipolar II, and cyclothymic disorder. Individuals with bipolar I disorder have at least one manic episode, whereas those with bipolar II disorder have at least one hypomanic episode and one melancholy episode. Cyclothymic disorder is a weaker type of bipolar disorder marked by less intense episodes of hypomanic and melancholy symptoms than bipolar I or II disorder.

Bipolar Disorder Symptoms

Bipolar disorder signs can differ based on the sort of bipolar disorder and the intensity of the symptoms. Among the most prevalent signs of bipolar illness are:

-**Mania**: -Excessive energy and activity -Extremely high self-esteem -The lower need for slumber -Racing ideas and fast speaking -Excessive impulsivity and risk-taking habits

-**Depression:** a sense of sadness or hopelessness -a loss of interest in pursuits -changes in eating and sleep habits -Fatigue and poor energy -Difficulty focusing -Suicide ideas

Bipolar Disorder Diagnosis

Many of the signs of bipolar disorder coincide with those of other mental health disorders, such as sadness and anxiety. A thorough psychiatric assessment, including a review of the individual's medical history and a talk of their symptoms with a mental health expert, is usually used to make a diagnosis.

Treatment and Coping Methods

Bipolar illness has no solution, but there are therapies and coping techniques that can help people control their symptoms and enhance their quality of life.

Mood stabilizers such as lithium and antipsychotics are frequently given to treat the signs of bipolar disorder. Psychotherapy, such as cognitive-behavioral treatment, can also assist with disease management and coping skills.

Lifestyle changes can also help manage the signs of bipolar illness. These can include frequent exercise, a nutritious diet, calming methods such as yoga or meditation, and obtaining enough sleep.

Individuals with bipolar disorder should collaborate closely with their mental health experts to create a customized therapy strategy that works for them. Individuals with bipolar disorder can control their symptoms and live happy lives with the proper therapy and coping techniques.

Amanda's Story: Riding the Rollercoaster of Mania and Depression

Amanda had always been a vibrant and imaginative individual. She enjoyed painting, writing, and traveling to new locations. However, as she approached her late adolescence, she started to experience extreme mood changes that would send her on a tumultuous journey of insanity and despair.

Amanda felt indestructible during her frenzied periods. She would create and write all night, take impromptu excursions to exotic locations, and spend money without hesitation. She believed she could accomplish anything and that nothing could deter her.

However, once the maniac high wore off, Amanda would sink into a profound melancholy. She'd feel helpless, unimportant, and as if nothing she did matter. She gave up drawing and writing and spent the majority of her days in bed, unable to muster the motivation to do anything.

Amanda wasn't identified with bipolar illness until she was in her twenties. She started to comprehend her situation and learn how to control her symptoms with the assistance of a mental health expert.

Amanda began taking medicine to control her emotions and undergoing counseling to learn coping skills. She also changed her lifestyle, such as having enough sleep, consuming a nutritious diet, and abstaining from narcotics and drinking.

Amanda's bipolar illness was not always simple to manage. She would occasionally neglect to take her medicine or revert to old behaviors. But she learned to identify the symptoms of hyperactivity and melancholy and would seek assistance when she needed it.

Amanda was able to achieve a feeling of equilibrium in her life over time. She continued to create and write, but in a more controlled manner, knowing that pushing herself too hard could result in a frenzied attack. She also learned to be gentle with herself during melancholy periods, understanding that they would pass.

Amanda's path with bipolar illness has been a wild trip, but she has emerged with a better knowledge of herself and her condition. She has discovered that controlling bipolar illness is a continuous process, but with the proper tools and support, she can navigate the ups and downs with greater comfort.

Robert's Story: The Highs and Lows of Living with Bipolar

Robert's tale exemplifies the ups and downs of life with bipolar illness. He has gone through times of intense exhilaration and inventiveness, as well as profound despair and futility.

Robert was always an imaginative kid as a toddler. He enjoyed drawing, writing tales, and playing instruments. He did, however, have strong emotional changes that were challenging to control. He'd go from feeling on top of the world to being profoundly depressed and uninspired in the blink of an eye.

Robert's emotional fluctuations became more severe as he grew older, and he was ultimately labeled with bipolar illness. He fought the prognosis and the thought of taking medicine at first, but after a few severe incidents, he recognized he needed assistance.

Robert has experienced many ups and downs over the years. He has felt unstoppable at moments, brimming with inventive energy and ideas. He would compose for hours, produce gorgeous work, and feel on top of the universe during these times. These highs, however, would be followed by times of profound sadness and hopelessness. During these lows, Robert found it difficult to get out of bed, consume, or even care for himself.

Despite these obstacles, Robert has persisted. He has learned to control his condition through medicine, counseling, and the help of friends and family. He has also discovered good avenues for his artistic energy, such as writing and singing.

Living with bipolar illness is difficult, but Robert's tale demonstrates that it is possible to flourish despite the difficulties. It is possible to handle the highs and lows of bipolar illness and live a happy life with the proper help and resources.

Lisa's Story: Coping with the Challenges of Rapid Cycling

Lisa is a 35-year-old lady who suffers from fast cyclical bipolar illness. Rapid cycling is a bipolar disorder subgroup marked by four or more bouts of mania or sadness in a calendar year. This means Lisa's emotions fluctuate quickly, sometimes within a day or even within hours.

It can be difficult to live with a fast-shifting bipolar illness. Lisa frequently describes herself as being on an emotional journey, with intense highs and lows that can be difficult to handle.

She feels like she can overcome the world when she is in a euphoric period, with limitless energy and excitement. But when she has a melancholy spell, she can hardly get out of bed, and everything seems useless.

Despite these difficulties, Lisa has evolved coping strategies that assist her in managing her situation. One of the most essential things she does is monitor her emotions and pinpoint the causes of mood changes. She has discovered that a shortage of sleep is a frequent cause of bipolar periods, so she attempts to keep a regular sleep routine.

Lisa has also built a solid network of friends and family who comprehend her situation and are available to her when she needs them. She sees a counselor who assists her in processing her feelings and developing coping techniques for her mood fluctuations. She also takes medication to assist with emotional stabilization, though she understands that medication alone is not a full answer.

Self-care is an essential part of Lisa's survival approach. She prioritizes things that bring her pleasure and leisure, such as literature, meditation, and spending time with family and friends. She also uses awareness and meditation to help her remain present at the moment and prevent getting caught up in her emotions.

Living with fast-cycling bipolar illness can be challenging, but Lisa's experience demonstrates that effective coping strategies can be developed and a happy life can be led. Lisa has found a way to handle her condition and flourish despite its difficulties by monitoring her emotions, developing a strong support system, emphasizing self-care, and working with mental health experts.

Chapter 4: Struggling with Schizophrenia

Schizophrenia is a serious and persistent mental disease that affects a person's thoughts, feelings, and behavior. Delusions, dreams, disordered speech, or behavior are common signs of schizophrenia, as are negative symptoms such as mental emptiness or retreat. These signs can be upsetting and distracting, making everyday living challenging for individuals with schizophrenia.

Living with schizophrenia can be difficult for both the individual suffering from the condition and their loved ones. Symptoms can be unexpected, and treatment may include a mix of medicine, counseling, and psychological support. Here are some of the most prevalent difficulties that individuals with schizophrenia may face:

Stigma: Schizophrenia is stigmatized, and individuals with the condition may experience prejudice and unfavorable views from others. This makes it difficult for them to seek assistance or participate in social activities, which can lead to seclusion and loneliness.

Medication adverse effects: Antipsychotic medicines, which are commonly used to treat schizophrenia, can cause weight increase, lethargy, and mobility problems. These adverse effects can be unpleasant and contribute to noncompliance with drug regimes.

Difficulty with social interactions: People with schizophrenia may struggle with social interactions, which can contribute to relationship problems and social alienation. They may have trouble comprehending social signals or articulating themselves, resulting in confusion and mistakes.

Financial problems: Schizophrenia can make it difficult to keep a job or finish school objectives, resulting in financial problems. This can exacerbate the tension and difficulties of coping with the condition.

Co-occurring disorders: People with schizophrenia may also have co-occurring disorders such as melancholy or drug misuse, which can make therapy and rehabilitation more difficult.

Regardless of these obstacles, it is critical to recall that individuals with schizophrenia can and do rehabilitate. Many individuals with schizophrenia can control their symptoms and live happy lives with the proper therapy and assistance. It is critical to obtain assistance as soon as feasible and to collaborate with a team of healthcare experts to create a personalized therapy strategy. lives. It is critical to obtain assistance as soon as feasible and to collaborate with a team of healthcare experts to create a personalized therapy strategy.

Tom's Story: Living with Hallucinations and Delusions

Tom's tale is a moving illustration of the difficulties that people suffering from dreams and illusions can encounter daily. Tom's experience with mental health problems began in his early twenties when he began to have intense and terrifying dreams that he couldn't explain. These dreams gradually took over his life, and he found himself increasingly secluded and detached from the world around him.

As Tom's health deteriorated, he started to have illusions, making it even more difficult for him to operate in his everyday life. He would become persuaded that people were tracking him, that the government was watching him, and that outside powers were controlling his thinking. These illusions exacerbated his worry and fear, and he found it difficult to trust anyone around him.

Despite his difficulties, Tom refused to give up optimism and sought assistance from mental health experts who could help him handle his symptoms. He started taking medicine to manage his dreams and illusions, and he also began taking counseling to address the deeper problems that had added to his condition.

Tom's symptoms gradually improved, and he was able to begin rebuilding his life. He reunited with friends and family members, found employment he liked, and even resumed his pastimes and interests. While he still had hallucinations and delusions on occasion, he was able to manage them effectively and keep them from taking over his life.

Living with dreams and illusions can be extremely challenging, but it is possible to handle these conditions and find a way forward. People like Tom can learn to deal with their situation and reclaim charge of their lives with the proper help and therapy.

Maria's Story: Battling the Stigma of Mental Illness

Maria's tale is one of fortitude, bravery, and persistence in the face of shame associated with mental disease. Maria was identified with bipolar disorder as a young woman in her mid-20s, a disease that produces intense mood fluctuations ranging from euphoric highs to despondent lows. While Maria battled to accept her prognosis, she was also subjected to the judgment and stupidity of those around her.

Despite the difficulties, Maria refused to let her illness define her. Instead, she embarked on a path of self-discovery and healing, enlisting the help of family, friends, and mental health professionals. She took medicine to control her symptoms, went to counseling, and acquired coping skills to help her cope with the ups and downs of her illness.

Despite all of this help, Maria encountered censure from people who did not comprehend her situation. She had been described as "crazy," "unstable," and "unpredictable." Some people even refused to interact with her because they were afraid her sickness would spread or that she would hurt them.

Maria refused to be discouraged by these pessimistic views. Instead, she became a mental health champion, speaking out about her experiences and confronting common myths about mental illness. She told her experience on social media, spoke with friends and family, and worked for mental health groups.

Maria's attempts to promote consciousness were successful, and she discovered that people were more tolerant and sympathetic than she had anticipated. She was also able to make other people suffering from mental illnesses feel less alone and more emboldened to seek assistance and support.

Maria's tale serves as a warning that mental disease is not a sign of frailty and that people suffering from mental illnesses deserve respect, support, and understanding. It is up to all of us to remove the shame associated with mental disease and build a more caring and open community.

Daniel's Story: Navigating the Complexities of Treatment and Recovery

Daniel's Story is a compelling illustration of the difficulties that people experience while managing the intricacies of therapy and rehabilitation. It emphasizes the significance of individualized, complete treatment that tackles each individual's distinct requirements.

Daniel's path started with an addiction, which led to a pattern of addiction, recidivism, and, eventually, legal problems. Despite several efforts to stop using narcotics, he found himself trapped in a downhill cycle, unable to break free from addiction's grasp.

He didn't start making headway in his rehabilitation until he got assistance from a thorough therapy program. This program offered him a variety of services, such as medical cleansing, individual and group counseling, and assistance with co-occurring mental health problems.

Even with the assistance of this software, Daniel encountered numerous obstacles along the road. He faced obstacles, battled the mental toll of addiction and rehabilitation, and had to negotiate a complicated system of insurance coverage and therapy choices.

Despite these challenges, Daniel persisted, relying on his resolve and the love and support of his loved ones to continue on the road to rehabilitation. He found fortitude in the relationships he formed with other people in recovery and learned to rely on them for support during challenging moments.

Daniel's path showed the value of individualized, thorough treatment that meets the unique requirements of each person in rehabilitation. He also demonstrated the importance of fortitude, tenacity, and a strong support structure in obtaining and keeping abstinence.

Overall, Daniel's Story serves as a potent lesson that treatment is a complicated and difficult process, but it is possible to conquer addiction and live a happy, clean life with the proper tools and support.

Chapter 5: Coping with Trauma and PTSD

Tragedy can leave profound mental wounds that require time and effort to recover. Post-stressful Stress Disorder (PTSD) is a psychiatric disorder that can arise as a result of observing or enduring a stressful incident. PTSD can result in strong and prolonged upsetting symptoms that have a substantial effect on a person's everyday living. However, coping with stress and PTSD and regaining a feeling of control and well-being is doable.

Understand PTSD: Understanding PTSD is the first step toward dealing with it. PTSD is a normal reaction to a stressful incident, not an indication of frailty or failure. Flashbacks, dreams, intrusive thoughts, denial, and hypervigilance are all signs of PTSD. These signs can have an impact on everyday living and interactions.

Seek expert assistance: PTSD is a curable disease, and getting professional help can help you heal significantly faster. PTSD symptoms can be alleviated with counseling and medicine from mental health experts. Cognitive-behavioral therapy (CBT) is an effective treatment for PTSD that can assist people in processing and managing their trauma-related feelings and ideas.

Create a helpful network: It is critical to have a network of family and friends who can offer mental support and empathy. Support organizations can also be useful in interacting with others who have encountered comparable stress and can provide a feeling of community and empathy.

Take care of your physical health: Trauma can harm your physical health, so it is critical to emphasize self-care. Eating a healthy diet, getting enough sleep, and exercising daily can all help to decrease tension and enhance general well-being.

Self-compassion: Coping with stress and PTSD can be difficult, and it is critical to be kind and sympathetic to oneself. It is acceptable to take time to recover and to recognize the success made along the road.

Relaxation methods, such as deep breathing, meditation, and yoga, can aid in stress management and the reduction of PTSD symptoms. These methods can also help you feel more at ease and relaxed.

Setting reasonable objectives can help you recover a feeling of control and achievement. It is critical to split objectives down into smaller, more manageable stages and to recognize success along the way.

To summarize, dealing with trauma and PTSD can be a difficult and continuing process, but it is possible to recover control and well-being. Seeking expert assistance, developing a support network, maintaining bodily health, exercising self-compassion, participating in calming methods, and establishing reasonable objectives are all important stages in dealing with trauma and PTSD. Individuals can heal from the mental wounds of tragedy and lead satisfying lives with time, tolerance, and support.

Emily's Story: Healing from the Wounds of War

Emily's tale is one of persistence, fortitude, and the restorative force of nature. Emily, a former fighter, had spent years in a warzone helping her nation. However, upon her return home, she discovered that the wounds of conflict extended far beyond the battleground.

Emily, like many soldiers, had been profoundly impacted by her wartime experiences. She was suffering from post-traumatic stress disorder (PTSD) signs such as dreams, flashbacks, and extreme worry. Emily struggled to interact with others and frequently felt alienated and alone.

Emily refused to give up in the face of adversity. She found assistance and started working with a PTSD-specialized psychiatrist. Emily discovered coping techniques in counseling that helped her handle her conditions and take charge of her life.

Emily found the strength of collaboration as well. She joined a veteran's support group, where she met others who had gone through comparable experiences. They shared their experiences, gave each other support, and assisted one another in navigating the difficulties of recovering from battle scars.

Emily's perseverance paid off in the end. She started to feel more linked to others as well as to her sense of mission. She discovered a new purpose in her life and started following her interests in painting and writing. Emily even began working for groups that assisted other survivors in healing from their tragedies.

Emily's tale shows that recovery is possible even in the face of enormous obstacles. Individuals can find the fortitude to surmount even the most challenging situations with the proper help and tools. They can also encourage others to find hope and recovery in their own lives by sharing their experiences.

Jake's Story: Finding Peace After a Tragic Loss

Jake's tale demonstrates the strength of fortitude and the human spirit's ability to surmount even the most adversity. It is a tale about finding purpose and calm during an unfathomable tragedy.

Jake was an accomplished entrepreneur, spouse, and parent of two children. He had a lovely house, a devoted family, and a bright future. But everything changed one day. His wife and children were killed in a terrible automobile mishap. Jake was abandoned, damaged, and destroyed.

Jake battled for months to come to terms with his loss. He cut himself off from the rest of the world, wallowing in sorrow and misery. He couldn't find significance or purpose in his existence any longer. His days were dominated by nothingness and suffering.

But Jake recognized one day that he couldn't keep living this way. Even in their absence, he knew his family would want him to live a joyful and satisfying existence. So he decided to take control of his life and find a path forward.

Jake sought expert assistance and found comfort in counseling. He gradually started to open up and express his emotions to others. He began working at a local charitable organization, where he discovered a new sense of meaning in assisting others in need. He started meditating, exercising frequently, and paying attention to his health and well-being.

Jake discovered that his anguish had lessened over time, and he was able to find serenity in his spirit. He came to understand that life is uncertain and that sad events do occur. But he also understood that he could choose how he would react to these occurrences.

Jake's tale serves as a lesson that there is always promise, even in the darkest of circumstances. Finding serenity after a catastrophe requires bravery and perseverance, but it is doable. Reaching out for assistance, finding a new purpose, and taking care of oneself can help one rediscover serenity and meaning in life.

Rachel's Story: Overcoming the Aftermath of Abuse

Rachel's tale exemplifies the perseverance and power of the human soul. She had endured years of violence at the hands of her father, and even after fleeing, she battled to surmount the anguish and agony she had endured.

But Rachel refused to let her past define her, and she started the process of mending and reconstructing her life with the aid of counseling and the support of loved ones.

One of the most difficult obstacles Rachel encountered was relearning to trust others. She found it difficult to open up to anyone, even those closest to her, after years of being deceived by someone she should have been able to trust completely. Rachel was able to gradually let down her defenses and establish healthy, important connections with the kindness and understanding of her counselor and loved ones.

Rachel also had to learn to respect and care for herself, which was never emphasized in her violent home. She learned the value of self-care in counseling and started to emphasize her wants and goals.

One of the most difficult parts of Rachel's path was facing the humiliation and remorse she had held for so long. She had been trained to think that the violence was her responsibility, that she had caused it. However, through counseling, she was able to see that the fault was entire with her attacker and that she was not to blame for his actions.

Rachel is doing well these days. She has a solid network of friends and family who adore and embrace her for who she is. She is following her dreams and enjoying life on her terms. Her history will always be a part of her, but she refuses to let it define her.

Rachel's tale is a potent reflection of the human spirit's fortitude, as well as the significance of getting assistance and support when we need it. We can surmount even the most challenging situations and live satisfying, happy lives with time, fortitude, and a desire to face our suffering.

Conclusion

Broken Minds, Broken Lives is a novel that presents a compilation of personal accounts from individuals who have contended with mental disease. The book seeks to break down the stigma surrounding the mental disease by sharing the real-life experiences of those impacted.

The accounts in the book address a variety of mental health problems, including melancholy, anxiety, bipolar disorder, and schizophrenia. Each narrative provides a distinct perspective on the difficulties and impediments encountered by individuals with mental disease, as well as the effect on their families and loved ones.

Overall, the novel is a forceful reminder that mental disease is a significant problem that impacts millions of people worldwide. By sharing these experiences, the book serves to increase consciousness and decrease the stigma associated with mental disease.

herbalism and naturopathic medication.

C. Modern Applications

Homegrown medication keeps on being a significant piece of numerous medical care frameworks all over the planet and is utilized for an extensive variety of ailments. In present-day times, homegrown cures are in many cases utilized related to regular clinical medicines as a corresponding treatment, to assist with overseeing side effects, decrease secondary effects, or backing by and large well-being and prosperity.

The absolute most normal purposes of natural medication today include:

Stomach-related issues: Numerous herbs are utilized to advance absorption and mitigate stomach related distresses, for example, bulging, gas, and acid reflux. Models incorporate ginger, peppermint, chamomile, and fennel.

Nervousness and stress: A few herbs have quiet and loosening properties that can assist with diminishing tension and stress. Models incorporate lavender, chamomile, passionflower, and valerian.

Agony and aggravation: Numerous herbs have mitigating and pain-relieving properties that can assist with decreasing torment and irritation. Models incorporate turmeric, ginger, boswellia, and white willow bark.

Invulnerable help: A few herbs are utilized to support the resistant framework and assist with forestalling sickness. Models incorporate echinacea, elderberry, and astragalus.

Ladies' well-being: Numerous herbs are utilized to help ladies' well-being and health, including directing periods, diminishing side effects of menopause, and supporting lactation. Models incorporate dark cohosh, red clover, and fenugreek.

While natural medication has a long history of purpose, it is essential to take note that not all herbs are protected or powerful for all individuals or all medical issues. It is critical to look for direction from certified medical care proficient before utilizing any natural cure, particularly if you have a previous ailment or are taking a prescription.

II. Types of Herbal Medicine

A. Traditional Chinese Medicine
Customary Chinese Medication (TCM) is a comprehensive medical care framework that has been polished in China for millennia. It depends on the standards of Qi (articulated "chee"), the fundamental energy that moves through the body, and the Yin-Yang hypothesis, which depicts the reciprocal and contradicting powers that exist in nature and the human body.
TCM incorporates many treatments, including needle therapy, homegrown medication, measuring,

moxibustion, and dietary treatment. One of the critical standards of TCM is equilibrium and agreement, and numerous TCM treatments are intended to assist with reestablishing harmony and concordance in the body to advance well-being and prosperity.

Needle therapy is one of the most notable and generally rehearsed treatments in TCM. It includes the inclusion of slight needles into explicit focuses on the body to invigorate the progression of Qi and advance recuperating. Needle therapy is in many cases used to treat a large number of conditions, including torment, stomach-related issues, nervousness, and fruitlessness.

Natural medication is one more significant part of TCM. TCM homegrown recipes are regularly a mix of a few herbs that cooperate to address an explicit medical issue. TCM specialists consider a patient's singular constitution and well-being history while recommending natural equations.

Measuring and moxibustion are two different treatments regularly utilized in TCM. Measuring includes the utilization of extraordinary cups that are put on the skin to make a pulling impact, which can assist with easing muscle pressure and advance mending. Moxibustion includes the consumption of a herb called mugwort close to needle therapy to invigorate the progression of Qi and advance recuperation.

Dietary treatment is likewise a significant part of TCM. In TCM, various food varieties are remembered to have various properties that can influence the body in various ways. TCM professionals might suggest explicit dietary changes or the utilization of specific herbs and enhancements to assist with supporting general well-being and health.

Today, TCM is drilled everywhere and is much of the time utilized related to regular clinical medicines to deal with an extensive variety of medical issues. While certain parts of TCM have been experimentally approved, others are as yet being considered, and the security and viability of numerous TCM treatments are not surely known. Likewise with any type of medical service, looking for direction from certified medical care proficient before utilizing any TCM therapy is significant

B. Ayurvedic Medication

Ayurvedic medication is an all-encompassing medical care framework that began in India quite a while back. It depends on the conviction that the psyche and body are interconnected and that the way to well-being and health lies in adjusting the body's three essential energies, or doshas: Vata, Pitta, and Kapha.

Ayurvedic medication incorporates a great many treatments, including homegrown medication, dietary treatment, yoga, reflection, back rub, and detoxification. One of the vital standards of Ayurveda is individualized treatment, and Ayurvedic specialists consider a patient's extraordinary constitution and well-being history while recommending medicines.

Homegrown medication is a significant part of Ayurvedic medication. Ayurvedic homegrown recipes are regularly a mix of a few herbs that cooperate to adjust the body's doshas and advance well-being and prosperity. Ayurvedic experts may likewise suggest explicit dietary changes, as well as the utilization of flavors and other culinary herbs, to assist with supporting by and large well-being.

Yoga and reflection are likewise significant parts of Ayurvedic medication. These practices are remembered to assist with adjusting the body and psyche, advance unwinding and stress decrease, and work on general well-being and prosperity.

Rub is one more ordinarily involved treatment in Ayurvedic medication. Ayurvedic knead procedures are intended to assist with advancing the progression of energy and eliminate blockages in the body, and may include the utilization of explicit oils and homegrown arrangements.

Detoxification is additionally a significant part of Ayurvedic medication. Ayurvedic professionals might suggest explicit dietary changes, as well as the utilization of herb and different treatments, to assist with eliminating poisons from the body and advance generally speaking well-being and health.

Today, Ayurvedic medication is drilled everywhere and is in many cases utilized related to ordinary clinical medicines to deal with an extensive variety of ailments. While certain parts of Ayurveda have been logically approved, others are as yet being examined, and the security and adequacy of numerous Ayurvedic treatments are not surely known. Likewise with any type of medical service, looking for direction from a certified medical service proficient before utilizing any Ayurvedic therapy is significant

C. Western Home grown Medication

Western homegrown medication, otherwise called herbalism or phytotherapy, is a type of medical care that utilizes plant-based prescriptions to advance the well-being and treat sickness. It has been utilized for millennia in Europe and different regions of the planet and has acquired prominence as of late as a reciprocal and elective treatment.

Western homegrown medication depends on the utilization of herb and other plant-based solutions to help the body's regular recuperating processes. Natural arrangements can take many structures, including teas, colors, cases, and creams.

Cultivators who practice Western homegrown medication might utilize many herbs to address different ailments. A few generally utilized herbs incorporate echinacea for invulnerable framework support, St. John's wort for misery and tension, and chamomile for stomach-related issues and a sleeping disorder.

Notwithstanding the utilization of herb, Western natural medication experts may likewise suggest dietary changes, way of life alterations, and other corresponding treatments to help in general well-being and prosperity.

Western homegrown medication is many times utilized in traditional clinical medicines and is for the most part viewed as protected when utilized under the direction of a certified medical services proficient. In any case, it is critical to take note that the security and viability of numerous homegrown cures have not been very much considered, and a few herb can communicate with prescriptions or cause secondary effects. Looking for direction from certified medical care proficient before utilizing any natural remedy is in this manner significant.

D. Native American Medicine

Local American medication, otherwise called customary Local American recuperating, is a comprehensive medical care framework that has been drilled by native people groups of North America for millennia. It depends on the conviction that the physical, mental, and profound parts of an individual are interconnected and that equilibrium and concordance are fundamental for good well-being.

Local American medication incorporates a large number of recuperating works, including homegrown medication, narrating, custom, dance, and supplication. The

utilization of herbs is a
significant part of Local
American medication, and
customary healers might
utilize many plants to address
different ailments.
One of the critical standards
of Local American medication
is individualized treatment.
Customary healers consider a
patient's novel constitution
and well-being history while
endorsing medicines, and
may likewise utilize divination
or other profound practices to
acquire an understanding of a
patient's well-being.
Notwithstanding the utilization
of herb and other normal
cures, Local American
medication likewise
accentuates the significance
of way of life factors like
eating routine, exercise, and
stress decrease. Customary
healers may likewise utilize
formal practices, for example,
sweat cabins and vision
missions to assist with
supporting generally speaking
well-being and prosperity.
Today, Local American
medication keeps on being

rehearsed by native networks across North America and is progressively perceived as an important type of medical service. Nonetheless, it is essential to take note that numerous parts of Local American medication have not been deductively approved, and the security and adequacy of a few conventional practices are not surely known. Likewise with any type of medical care, looking for direction from certified medical care proficient before utilizing any Local American cure or practice is significant.

III. How Herbal Medicine Works

A. Active Compounds

Homegrown meds contain a wide assortment of dynamic mixtures, which are liable for their helpful impacts. Probably the most widely recognized kinds of dynamic mixtures found in natural drugs include:

Alkaloids: These are nitrogen-containing intensifies tracked down in plants, and are in many cases answerable for their pharmacological impacts. Instances of alkaloids incorporate caffeine, nicotine, and morphine.

Flavonoids: These are a gathering of polyphenolic intensifiers that are known for their cell reinforcement and calming impacts. Flavonoids are found in a large number of plants, including citrus natural products, berries, and tea.

Terpenoids: These are a different gathering of mixtures tracked down in numerous rejuvenating ointments and saps, and are liable for the trademark smells of plants. Terpenoids are known for their calming, antiviral, and antifungal properties.

Glycosides: These are intensified that contain a sugar particle joined to a non-sugar particle. Glycosides are tracked down in many plants and are much of the time liable for their restorative impacts. Instances of glycosides incorporate cardiovascular glycosides, which are utilized to treat heart conditions, and saponins, which make antimicrobial and calming impacts.

Phenolic acids: These are a gathering of sweet-smelling acids that are tracked down in many plants, and are known for their cell reinforcement and mitigating impacts. Instances of phenolic acids incorporate caffeic corrosive and ferulic corrosive.

Tannins: These are a gathering of polyphenolic intensifies that are tracked down in many plants and are known for their astringent properties. Tannins are much of the time used to treat loose bowels and other stomach-related issues.

The particular dynamic mixtures found in homegrown drugs can change generally contingent upon the plant species, the piece of the plant utilized, and the strategy for planning. While numerous homegrown cures have been utilized for a long time, the security and viability of a few natural prescriptions are not surely known, and looking for direction from a certified medical care proficient before utilizing any natural remedy is significant

B. Instruments of Activity

Homegrown meds work through various systems of activity, contingent upon the particular dynamic mixtures and the condition being dealt with. Probably the most well-known systems of activity for homegrown prescriptions include:

Tweaking catalyst movement: Numerous homegrown drugs contain intensifiers that can cooperate with compounds in the body, either restraining or enacting them. For instance, St. John's wort contains hyperforin and hypericin, which are remembered to hinder the reuptake of serotonin, dopamine, and norepinephrine, prompting an upper impact.

Cancer prevention agent impacts: Natural drugs that

contain flavonoids, phenolic acids, and other cancer prevention agent mixtures can assist with shielding the body's cells from oxidative harm, which is ensnared in an extensive variety of medical issues, including malignant growth and cardiovascular sickness.

Calming impacts: Numerous homegrown medications contain intensities that can assist with decreasing irritation in the body, which is critical considering numerous persistent sicknesses. For instance, curcumin, the dynamic compound in turmeric, makes powerful mitigating impacts and is utilized to treat a scope of fiery circumstances.

Safe tweak: A few homegrown medications, like echinacea, are remembered to invigorate the insusceptible framework, assisting with warding off diseases and backing generally invulnerable capability.

Balancing synapses: Certain natural drugs contain

intensities that can influence the degrees of synapses in the cerebrum, prompting changes in the state of mind and conduct. For instance, kava contains kavalactones, which make anxiolytic impacts and are utilized to treat nervousness.

Antimicrobial impacts: Numerous natural prescriptions contain intensities that have antimicrobial properties, which can assist with fending off diseases brought about by microbes, infections, and different microorganisms. These components of activity are only a couple of instances of the numerous ways that homegrown drugs can influence the body. The particular components of activity for a specific natural cure will rely upon the dynamic mixtures present in the plant and the condition being dealt with. It is essential to take note of that the security and viability of numerous homegrown cures have not been very much examined, and looking for direction from certified medical services proficient before utilizing any natural remedy is generally significant

C. Viability and Security

The viability and security of homegrown prescriptions can shift generally contingent upon the particular plant species, the piece of the plant utilized, the technique for planning, and the singular utilizing the cure. While numerous homegrown cures have been utilized for a long time and are by and large thought to be protected, a few natural prescriptions can connect with different meds, cause unfavorable impacts, or even be harmful.

Adequacy:

The adequacy of homegrown medications can be challenging to study, as many elements can impact their consequences for the body. While a few natural drugs have been very much contemplated and demonstrated to be successful for specific circumstances, others have not been concentrated thoroughly, and their viability stays questionable. It is vital to look for direction from certified medical care proficient before utilizing any natural solution to guarantee that it is suitable for the particular condition being dealt with.

Security:

The security of homegrown meds can likewise be hard to decide, as numerous natural cures contain dynamic mixtures that can interface with different drugs or cause unfavorable impacts. Some potential well-being concerns related to natural meds include:

Collaboration with drugs: A few natural cures can cooperate with professionally prescribed prescriptions, either by expanding or diminishing their belongings. For instance, St. John's wort can diminish the viability of specific meds, for example, conception prevention pills and a few antidepressants.

Unfavorable impacts: A few natural cures can cause unfriendly impacts, like gastrointestinal steamed, hypersensitive responses, or liver harm. For instance, high portions of kava can cause liver harm.

Tainting: Natural cures can be polluted with weighty metals, pesticides, or different poisons, which can be hurtful to well-being.

Misidentification: Natural cures that are not as expected can be perilous, as various plant species can contrastingly affect the body. For instance, a few types of plants intently look like noxious plants, and misidentification can prompt serious damage.

To limit the gamble of unfriendly impacts and guarantee the well-being and viability of homegrown cures, looking for direction from a certified medical service proficient before utilizing any natural remedy is significant. They can assist with guaranteeing that the natural medication is proper for the particular condition being dealt with, and can give direction on suitable doses, possible cooperation, and expected incidental effects

IV. Common Herbs and Their Uses

A. Chamomile
Chamomile is a well-known natural medication that has been utilized for quite a long time to treat many circumstances. It is obtained from the dried blossoms of the chamomile plant, which is an individual from the Asteraceae family. Chamomile is accessible in different structures, including teas, containers, and skin creams.
Utilizes:
Chamomile is regularly used to treat conditions, for example,
Tension and sleep deprivation: Chamomile meaningfully affects the body

and is ordinarily used to assist with advancing unwinding and decreasing nervousness and stress.

Stomach-related issues: Chamomile has antispasmodic properties, which can assist with diminishing squeezing and uneasiness in the gastrointestinal system. It is regularly used to treat conditions like heartburn, gas, and bulging.

Skin conditions: Chamomile has mitigating properties and is generally used to relieve and quiet bothered or aroused skin. It is normally used to treat conditions like skin inflammation, psoriasis, and skin inflammation.

Feminine spasms: Chamomile has antispasmodic properties and is generally used to assist with diminishing the force of feminine issues.

Wound recuperating: Chamomile has been displayed to have antimicrobial properties and can assist with advancing injury mending.

Security:
Chamomile is by and large viewed as protected when utilized as coordinated. In any case, certain individuals might be sensitive to chamomile, and unfavorably susceptible responses can go from gentle skin aggravation to additional serious side effects like hypersensitivity. Chamomile can likewise communicate for certain meds, like blood thinners and tranquilizers, and ought not to be utilized in blend with these drugs without direction from a certified medical services proficient. Pregnant ladies ought to likewise practice alert while utilizing chamomile, as it might expand the gamble of unsuccessful labor. Likewise, chamomile might have a gentle blood-diminishing impact and ought to be utilized with alertness by individuals with draining issues or those taking blood-diminishing drugs.
By and large, chamomile is a protected and compelling natural medication for various

circumstances when utilized suitably and under the direction of a certified medical services proficient
B. Echinacea
Echinacea is a famous homegrown medication that is gotten from the roots or more ground portions of the Echinacea plant, which is an individual from the daisy family. Echinacea is generally used to support the resistant framework and is accessible in different structures, including teas, containers, and concentrates.
Utilizes:
Echinacea is usually used to treat or forestall the normal cold, influenza, and other respiratory diseases. It is additionally used to treat conditions, for example,
Upper respiratory contaminations: Echinacea is regularly used to treat conditions like sore throat, bronchitis, and sinusitis.
Skin diseases: Echinacea has been displayed to have antibacterial and antifungal properties and is generally

used to treat skin contaminations like skin inflammation, bubbles, and abscesses.

Wound recuperating: Echinacea has been displayed to have mitigating properties and can assist with advancing injury mending.

Urinary lot diseases: Echinacea has been displayed to have antibacterial properties and might be successful in treating urinary plot contaminations.

Sensitivities: Echinacea might have allergy med properties and might be powerful in lessening the side effects of sensitivities.

Wellbeing: Echinacea is for the most part viewed as protected when utilized as coordinated. In any case, certain individuals might encounter gentle aftereffects, for example, stomach upset, sickness, or tipsiness. Unfavorably susceptible responses to echinacea are uncommon, however, can happen in certain people.

Echinacea may likewise connect for certain prescriptions, like immunosuppressants and certain antidepressants, and ought not to be utilized in a mix with these drugs without direction from certified medical care proficient.

By and large, echinacea is a protected and compelling natural medication for supporting the safe framework and treating various circumstances when utilized fittingly and under the direction of certified medical care proficient

C. Ginkgo Biloba

Ginkgo biloba is a well-known homegrown medication obtained from the leaves of the ginkgo tree. It has been utilized for quite a long time in conventional Chinese medication to treat different circumstances and is currently generally utilized all through the world. Ginkgo biloba is accessible in different structures, including cases, tablets, and concentrates. Utilizes:

Ginkgo biloba is ordinarily used to work on mental capability, memory, and fixation. It is likewise used to treat conditions, for example, Age-related mental degradation: Ginkgo biloba might be successful in working on mental capability and memory in more seasoned grown-ups.
Fringe vascular sickness: Ginkgo biloba has been displayed to further develop the bloodstream to the arms, legs, and mind, and might be successful in treating conditions like fringe vascular illness and Raynaud's sickness.
Tinnitus: Ginkgo biloba might be viable in decreasing the seriousness and recurrence of tinnitus (ringing in the ears).
Macular degeneration: Ginkgo biloba might be viable in easing back the movement of macular degeneration, a typical age-related eye condition.
Tension and wretchedness: Ginkgo biloba may have

gentle anxiolytic and stimulant impacts.

Security:

Ginkgo biloba is by and large viewed as protected when utilized as coordinated. In any case, certain individuals might encounter gentle aftereffects, for example, cerebral pain, stomach upset, or tipsiness. Ginkgo biloba may likewise communicate for certain drugs, like blood thinners and certain antidepressants, and ought not to be utilized in blend with these prescriptions without direction from a certified medical services proficient.

Pregnant and breastfeeding ladies ought to likewise try not to utilize ginkgo biloba, as its well-being has not been laid out in these populaces.

Generally, ginkgo biloba is a protected and powerful homegrown medication for working on mental capability and treating various circumstances when utilized fittingly and under the direction of certified medical care proficient.

D. St. John's Wort
St. John's wort is a well-known natural medication obtained from the blossoms and leaves of the St. John's wort plant. It has been utilized for a long time to treat various circumstances, including sorrow, uneasiness, and rest issues. St. John's wort is accessible in different structures, including containers, tablets, teas, and concentrates.

Utilizes:
St. John's wort is generally used to treat gently to direct misery and tension. It is additionally used to treat conditions, for example,
Occasional emotional problem (Miserable): St. John's wort might be viable in diminishing side effects of Miserable, a kind of gloom that happens throughout the cold weather months.
Rest issues: St. John's wort might be compelling in further developing rest quality and lessening the recurrence of rest aggravations.

Menopausal side effects: St. John's wort might be viable in decreasing the recurrence and seriousness of hot blazes and other menopausal side effects.

Nerve torment: St. John's wort might be powerful in decreasing nerve torment related to conditions like sciatica and shingles.

Wellbeing:

St. John's wort is for the most part viewed as protected when utilized as coordinated. Be that as it may, certain individuals might encounter gentle aftereffects like dry mouth, wooziness, or gastrointestinal bombshell. St. John's wort may likewise collaborate for certain prescriptions, for example, antidepressants, conception prevention pills, and blood thinners, and ought not to be utilized in mix with these meds without direction from certified medical care proficient.

St. John's wort ought not to be utilized by pregnant or breastfeeding ladies, as its wellbeing has not been laid out in these populaces.

By and large, St. John's wort is a protected and powerful natural medication for treating despondency, nervousness, and different circumstances when utilized fittingly and under the direction of a certified medical services proficient

E. Turmeric

Turmeric is a well-known homegrown medication that is gotten from the foundation of the turmeric plant, which is local to India and Southeast Asia. It has been utilized for quite a long time in conventional Ayurvedic medication to treat different circumstances and is presently broadly utilized all through the world. Turmeric is accessible in different structures, including cases, tablets, and concentrates.

Utilizes:

Turmeric is usually used to treat aggravation and agony and is known for its cell reinforcement properties. It is

additionally used to treat conditions, for example,
Joint inflammation: Turmeric might be successful in diminishing irritation and agony related to osteoarthritis and rheumatoid joint pain.
Stomach-related messes: Turmeric might be successful in diminishing side effects of stomach-related issues like provocative gut illness and bad-tempered gut condition.
Cardiovascular well-being: Turmeric might be powerful in diminishing the gamble of cardiovascular illness by further developing cholesterol levels and lessening irritation.
Skin wellbeing: Turmeric might be viable in further developing skin wellbeing and diminishing the indications of maturing.
Disease: Turmeric might have against malignant growth properties and might be powerful in forestalling or treating particular kinds of disease.
Security:
Turmeric is by and large viewed as protected when

utilized as coordinated. In any case, certain individuals might encounter gentle aftereffects like gastrointestinal irritation or unfavorably susceptible responses. Turmeric may likewise cooperate with certain drugs, like blood thinners and diabetes prescriptions, and ought not to be utilized in a mix with these meds without direction from a certified medical services proficient.

Pregnant and breastfeeding ladies ought to likewise try not to utilize turmeric, as its security has not been laid out in these populaces.

In general, turmeric is a protected and compelling homegrown medication for treating irritation, torment, and different circumstances when utilized suitably and under the direction of certified medical care proficient.

V. Herbal Preparations

A. Infusions

Mixtures are a typical strategy
for getting ready homegrown
meds, in which the dynamic
mixtures are removed from
the plant material by soaking
it in steaming hot water.
Mixtures are otherwise called
teas, and can be produced
using various herb and plants.
To make implantation, the
herbs or plant material is put
in a holder, for example, a tea
sifter or steeping ball, and
boiling water is poured ready
to be done. The blend is then
permitted to soak for a
specific timeframe, contingent
upon the plant material and
the strength of the mixture.
The soaking time can go from
a couple of moments to a few
hours.
Imbuements can be
consumed hot or cold and can
be improved with honey or
different sugars whenever
wanted. They can likewise be
joined with different herb and
plants to make more intricate
mixes and flavors.
Imbuements are usually used
to treat various
circumstances, like sleep

deprivation, nervousness, and stomach-related messes.
They are likewise utilized as a day-to-day tonic to advance general well-being and health. Mixtures are by and large safe when utilized as coordinated, yet can interface for certain drugs, so it is vital to talk with certified medical services proficient before utilizing them
B. Decoctions
Decoctions are a strategy for getting ready natural prescriptions that includes heating the plant material in water to separate the dynamic mixtures. Decoctions are ordinarily produced using harder, more stringy plant materials like roots, bark, and seeds.
To make a decoction, the plant material is set in a pot with cold water and heated to the point of boiling. The combination is then stewed for a while, normally somewhere in the range of 20 and an hour, to extricate the dynamic mixtures. The decoction is then stressed and the fluid is consumed.

Decoctions are regularly used to treat conditions like respiratory diseases, stomach-related messes, and feminine issues. They are likewise utilized as a day-to-day tonic to advance generally speaking well-being and health.

Decoctions are for the most part safe when utilized as coordinated, however, can cooperate for certain prescriptions, so it is vital to talk with certified medical services proficient before utilizing them. Since decoctions include heating the plant material for a lengthy time frame, they can likewise be less intense than different types of homegrown prescriptions, like concentrates or colors.

C. Colors

Colors are a concentrated type of natural medication that involves liquor or a combination of liquor and water as a dissolvable to extricate the dynamic mixtures from the plant material. Colors are much of the time utilized when a more powerful or dependable impact is wanted.

To make a color, the plant material is put in a container with liquor and water, and permitted to soak for a very long time to a while. During this time, the dynamic mixtures are separated from the plant material and break up into the liquor and water blend. The blend is then stressed, and the fluid is the color.

Colors are commonly taken orally by putting a couple of drops under the tongue, or by weakening them in water or squeezing. Colors can likewise be added to skin arrangements, like creams or treatments, for outer use. Colors are ordinarily used to treat conditions like tension, sleep deprivation, and stomach-related messes. They are likewise utilized as a day-to-day tonic to advance generally speaking well-being and health. Colors are by and large safe when utilized as coordinated, however, an interface for certain prescriptions, so it is critical to talk with certified medical care proficient before utilizing them.

D. Cases and Tablets

Cases and tablets are helpful types of natural medication that are broadly utilized because of their convenience and convenience. Containers and tablets are made by compacting or typifying a powdered type of herbs or plant material.

Cases are little, round, and hollow holders made of gelatin or a plant-based other option, and loaded up with powdered homegrown material. Cases are regularly gulped with water and are intended to disintegrate in the stomach, permitting the dynamic mixtures to be assimilated into the circulation system.

Tablets, then again, are compacted types of powdered natural material that may likewise contain fasteners, fillers, and other excipients. Tablets are additionally

commonly gulped with water
and are intended to break
down in the stomach.
Containers and tablets are
much of the time used to treat
conditions like agony,
aggravation, and safe
framework problems. They
are likewise utilized as a day-
to-day supplement to advance
general well-being and health.
Cases and tablets are for the
most part safe when utilized
as coordinated, however, can
cooperate for certain
prescriptions, so it is critical to
talk with certified medical care
proficient before utilizing
them. Containers and tablets
may likewise have different
retention rates and
bioavailability contrasted with
different types of homegrown
medication, like colors or
mixtures, so it is critical to pick
the fitting structure given the
ideal restorative impact

VI. Safety Considerations and Side Effects

A. Interactions with Medications

Homegrown meds can interface with a solution and non-prescription drugs, as well as with different herbs and enhancements. A portion of these collaborations can be destructive and can cause unfriendly impacts or decrease the viability of the medicine.

It is essential to illuminate your medical care supplier about any natural enhancements or cures you are taking, as well as any drugs you are presently taking or plan to take from now on. This data can help your medical services supplier to recognize likely cooperation and make fitting changes following your therapy plan.

A few homegrown meds can cooperate with prescriptions by influencing how the medicine is used or consumed in the body. For instance, St. John's wort can decrease the viability of specific meds, including antidepressants, anti-conception medication pills, and blood thinners.

Different herbs can associate with prescriptions by upgrading their belongings or expanding the gamble of secondary effects. For instance, Ginkgo biloba can expand the gamble of draining when taken with blood thinners and can improve the impacts of some upper drugs.

It is essential to take note that not all connections between homegrown meds and drugs are known or completely comprehended. Thus, it is essential to utilize alert while consolidating herb and drugs and to talk with certified medical services proficient before utilizing any homegrown cures or enhancements.

B. Unfriendly Responses

While homegrown meds are for the most part viewed as protected, they can in any case cause unfriendly responses in certain people. Antagonistic responses can go from gentle to serious and can change contingent upon the herbs or plant material, measurements, and individual factors like age, well-being status, and prescription use. A few normal unfriendly responses related to homegrown medication include:

Unfavorably susceptible responses: A few people might be oversensitive to specific herb or plant materials, and may encounter side effects like tingling, hives, or trouble relaxing.

Gastrointestinal side effects: A few natural medications can cause sickness, heaving, loose bowels, or other stomach-related side effects.

Liver poisonousness: Certain herbs, like kava and comfrey, have been related to liver harmfulness and ought to be utilized with an alert or kept away from through and through.

Corporations with drugs: As referenced prior, a few herbs can collaborate with prescriptions and cause unfavorable impacts or lessen their viability.
It is essential to take note that the quality and virtue of homegrown meds can differ, and defiled or debased items can build the gamble of unfriendly responses. To limit the gamble of antagonistic responses, it is vital to buy homegrown prescriptions from trustworthy sources and to painstakingly adhere to measurement and use directions.
On the off chance that you experience any unfavorable responses in the wake of utilizing a homegrown medication, you ought to quit utilizing it right away and talk with certified medical care proficient
C. Tainting and Quality Control
Tainting and absence of value control are significant worries in the creation and utilization of homegrown medications.

Tainting can happen because of elements like ill-advised reaping and stockpiling, utilization of pesticides and different synthetic substances, or unintentional pollution during handling or assembling.

Natural medications can likewise be dependent upon defilement, where substandard or non-home-grown materials are added to the item, or replacement, where one herb is filled in for another. Defilement and replacement can prompt off-base marking and can think twice about the well-being and adequacy of the item.

To guarantee the well-being and nature of homegrown drugs, it is critical to buy items from trustworthy sources that have thorough quality control estimates set up. Quality control measures might incorporate testing for pollutants like weighty metals, pesticides, and microorganisms, as well as confirming the legitimacy and virtue of the herbs or plant material.

As well as buying from trustworthy sources, it is essential to adhere to measurement and utilization directions cautiously and to talk with certified medical care proficient before utilizing any natural cures or enhancements. Medical services experts can give direction on suitable use and can assist recognize possible dangers and communications with prescriptions.

VII. Future Directions and Research

A. Emerging Trends in Herbal Medicine

There are a few arising patterns in natural medication that are acquiring prominence and consideration lately. A portion of these patterns include:

Natural enhancements for mental wellbeing: There is developing interest in the utilization of homegrown supplements, for example, ginkgo biloba and Bacopa monnieri, for working on mental capability and memory.

Weed-based cures: With the rising sanctioning of marijuana for clinical and sporting use, there is developing interest in the utilization of pot-based cures, for example, CBD oil, for an assortment of medical issues, including torment, nervousness, and rest problems.

Adaptogenic herb: Adaptogenic herb, for example, ashwagandha and Rhodiola, are herbs that are remembered to assist the body with adjusting to pressure and work on general flexibility and prosperity.

Natural solutions for stomach wellbeing: There is developing acknowledgment of the significance of stomach well-being for generally speaking well-being and prosperity, and there is expanding interest in the utilization of homegrown cures, for example, licorice root and tricky elm, for advancing stomach-related wellbeing.

Customized natural medication: With propels in innovation and hereditary testing, there is expanding interest in the utilization of customized homegrown medication, where homegrown cures are custom-made to a singular's remarkable hereditary cosmetics and well-being needs.

These arising patterns feature the developing interest in homegrown medication and the potential for new and imaginative ways to deal with medical care utilizing normal cures. Nonetheless, it means quite a bit to proceed to study and research the well-being and viability of these arising patterns to guarantee that they are protected and powerful for boundless use

B. Clinical Preliminaries and Proof-Based Medication

Clinical preliminaries are a significant method for laying

out the well-being and adequacy of homegrown medications. Proof put together medication depends concerning all on planned clinical preliminaries that observe thorough logical guidelines to give solid and reproducible outcomes. Clinical preliminaries can assist with distinguishing the ideal measurements, definitions, and courses of organization for homegrown meds, as well as recognize likely aftereffects and medication connections. There are a few difficulties related to directing clinical preliminaries for homegrown medications, remembering the changeability for the quality and power of the plant material utilized in the preliminaries, as well as the intricacy and fluctuation of the dynamic mixtures present in the plant material. Moreover, there are many times an absence of financing for clinical preliminaries of homegrown medications, which can make it hard to lead huge-scope preliminaries with adequate measurable power.

Notwithstanding these difficulties, there has been expanding interest in leading very much-planned clinical preliminaries for natural medications, and a few top-notch examinations have been conducted lately. For instance, a randomized controlled preliminary of St. John's wort observed that the herb was powerful in treating gentle to direct melancholy, while an orderly survey of clinical preliminaries of echinacea observed that the herb was viable in lessening the length and seriousness of cold side effects.

By and large, the proof base for homegrown medication is developing, and there is expanding acknowledgment of the significance of integrating proof-based natural medication into medical services practice. Nonetheless, it means a lot to keep on leading thorough clinical preliminaries and to utilize proof-based rules to guarantee the protected and compelling utilization of natural drugs in clinical practice.

C. Combination with Traditional Medication

There is a developing interest in the combination of natural medication with ordinary medication. This approach is some of the time alluded to as integrative medication or correlative and elective medication (CAM). The objective of integrative medicine is to give a comprehensive way to deal with patient consideration that joins the best of traditional and reciprocal treatments. Integrative medication perceives the expected advantages of homegrown medication, while likewise perceiving the significance of proof-based medication and well-being principles. Integrative medication specialists ordinarily work intimately with traditional medical services suppliers to guarantee that patients get

protected and successful
therapy that is customized to
their singular necessities.
There are multiple manners
by which homegrown
medication can be
coordinated with ordinary
medication. For instance,
homegrown drugs can be
utilized related to physician-
endorsed meds to upgrade
the helpful impacts of the
prescriptions or to diminish
incidental effects. Moreover,
homegrown meds can be
utilized as an essential
treatment choice for specific
circumstances, for example,
gentle to direct
discouragement or
nervousness.
There are additionally a few
difficulties related to the
combination of natural
medication and customary
medication. For instance,
there might be
communications between
natural drugs and doctor-
prescribed prescriptions that
can prompt antagonistic
impacts. Moreover, there
might be contrasts in the way

to deal with treatment between customary medication and homegrown medication, which can make it challenging to track down a typical way to deal with patient consideration. Notwithstanding these difficulties, there is a developing acknowledgment of the likely advantages of integrative medication and the significance of a comprehensive way to deal with patient considerations. Thus, numerous medical services suppliers are progressively open to coordinating natural medication into their training, and there are currently a few integrative medication facilities that offer a great many corresponding treatments, including homegrown medication.

www.ingramcontent.com/pod-product-compliance
Lightning Source LLC
Chambersburg PA
CBHW071025260726
48662CB00024B/2000